QUIT DRINKING

The Complete Guide on Quitting Alcohol & Be Sober
For Life

By Elliott J. Power

Legal & Disclaimer

2

periodically made to this book as and when needed. Where appropriate and necessary, you must consult a professional (including but not limited to your doctor, attorney, financial advisor, or such other professional advisor) before using any of the suggested remedies, techniques, or information in this book.

Upon using the contents and information contained in this book, you agree to hold harmless the Author from and against any damages, costs, and expenses, including any legal fees potentially resulting from the application of any of the information provided by this book. This disclaimer applies to any loss, damages or injury caused by the use and application, whether directly or indirectly, of any advice or information presented, whether for breach of contract, tort, negligence, personal injury, criminal intent, or under any other cause of action.

You agree to accept all risks of using the information presented inside this book.

You agree that by continuing to read this book, where appropriate and necessary, you shall consult a professional (including but not limited to your doctor, attorney, or financial advisor or such other advisor as needed) before using any of the suggested remedies, techniques, or information in this book.

TABLE OF CONTENTS

Chapter 1: HOW TO BREAK A BAD HABIT (AND REPLACE

IT WITH A GOOD ONE)

Poor habits are interrupting your life and preventing you from reaching your goals. They put your safety at risk-both psychologically and physically. And they are wasting your time and your energy. Why are we even doing them, then? And most importantly, will you do something about it?

I've written before about the science of how behaviors develop, so let's now concentrate on the practice of making real-world changes. How do you eradicate your negative habits and then stick to healthy ones? I still don't have all the answers but keep reading, and I'm going to share what I've heard about breaking a bad habit.

What causes bad habits?

Two things trigger most of your bad habits ... stress and boredom. Bad habits are, most of the time, simply a way to cope with tension and boredom. It can be an easy answer to stress and boredom, from chewing your nails to overspending on a shopping spree to drinking every weekend to wasting time on the internet.

Yet that shouldn't be the way it is. You should teach yourself new and healthier ways to cope with stress and depression, which you can replace those bad habits. Of course, frequently, the underlying problems trigger the tension or frustration that is on the surface. These issues can be hard to think about, but if you are serious about making changes, you must be honest with yourself.

Are there any convictions or explanations behind the poor habit? Is there anything more profound — a fear, an occurrence, or a limiting belief — that causes you to hang on to something bad for you? To conquer this, it is important to consider the causes of bad habits.

You're not eliminating a bad habit; you are replacing it.

All the habits you have right now — whether good or bad — are for a reason in your life. These behaviors provide you with a benefit somehow, even if they are otherwise bad for you.

The gain is often psychological, as it is with smoking or drugs. Even when you live in a relationship that's terrible for you, it's miserable. And your bad behavior is, in many

situations, an easy way to cope with stress. For example, you can bite your nails, pull your hair, tap your foot or clench your jaw.

These "benefits" or explanations often refer to minor bad habits.

Opening your email inbox, for example, as soon as you turn on your computer might make you feel linked. Looking at all those emails simultaneously kills your efficiency, splits your focus, and overwhelms you with tension. No, it doesn't make you feel like you're "missing out," ... and so you do it again. Since bad habits have some form of benefit in your life, it's really hard to just remove them. (This is why simple advice such as ', please stop doing it' never works.)

You will then substitute a bad habit with a new habit that

offers similar value. For example, if you smoke when you get stressed, then when that happens, it's a bad plan to "just stop smoking" Instead of smoking a cigarette, you should come up with a better way to cope with stress and introduce the new behavior.

In other words, bad habits answer some of your life's needs. So, it's easier for that reason to replace your bad habits with a healthy activity that serves the same need. If you just plan to cut bad habits without replacing them, you will have some unmet needs, and it will be hard to adhere to a "just don't do it" routine for a long time.

HOW TO BREAK A BAD HABIT

Below are some helpful suggestions to break your bad habits and focus on the process in your way.

1.Choose a substitute for your bad habit. You need to have a plan in advance for how you'll respond when facing the stress or boredom that prompts your bad habits. What will you do when you are getting the urge to smoke? (Example: use breathing exercises.)

What do you do when Facebook is making you dawdle?

(Example: write a paragraph for work.) Whatever it is and whatever you're struggling with, you need to have a plan for what you're going to do, rather than your bad habit.

2.Cut the maximum number of stimuli available. If you smoke when you're drinking, do not go to the lounge. If you are in the house eating cookies, then throw them all away. If the first thing you do is pick up the TV remote when you sit on the sofa, then hide the remote in a separate space in the wardrobe. Make it easier to break bad habits in yourself by avoiding the things that cause them.

3.Join hands with someone else. So how much do you want to take a private diet? And maybe you're "quitting smoking," ... but you've kept it to yourself? (No one will see you fail that way, right?) Instead, pair up with somebody and quit. The two of you should keep each other accountable and celebrate your victories. Knowing others expect you to be better is a powerful motivator.

4.Surround yourself with people living the way you

want to be living. You don't have to cut off your old friends but don't underestimate the ability to discover new ones.

5.Visualize yourself effectively. Watch yourself throw away the cigarettes or buy healthy food or wake up early. Whatever the bad habit is that you're trying to smash, kill it, smile and enjoy your success. See how you develop a new identity.

6.You don't have to be someone; you just have to return to the old you. So often, we assume that we have to become entirely new people to break our bad habits. The reality is you have it in yourself to be someone without your bad habits. It's just doubtful that you've had these bad habits all of your life. You don't have to quit smoking; you just have to go back to being a non-smoker. You don't have to turn yourself into a good person; you just need to get back to being a good person. Even if it was years ago, you've lived without this bad habit, which means you can do it again, most certainly.

7.Using the term "but" to practice negative self-talk. One thing about fighting bad habits is punishing yourself for not behaving better. It's easy to tell yourself how bad you feel each time you mess up or make a mistake. Whenever this occurs, put "but" in the sentence.

•"I'm overweight and out of shape, but a few months from now, I will be in shape."

•"I'm dumb, and no one respects me, so I'm learning to improve user skills."

•"I'm a failure, but sometimes everyone fails."

8.Plan for failure. Now and then, we mess everyone up. And prepare for it rather than beating yourself up over a mistake. We all get off course; what distinguishes top performers from everyone else is that they very easily get back on track. Read this article for various tactics that will help you come back when you make a mistake.

Where to go from here

If you are looking for the first step to break your bad habits, I suggest that you start with knowledge. The way you feel about your bad habits is easy to get caught up in.

You may feel guilty or waste your time thinking of how you want things to be ... but these feelings take you away from what is going on.

It's understanding that will show you how progress can be made.

•Really, when does your bad habit happen?

•How often do you do it every day?

•Where are you from?

•What are you?

•What triggers and causes the behavior to take off?

Only monitoring these issues will increase your knowledge of the conduct and give you thousands of ideas to stop it.

It takes time and energy to break bad habits, but also it takes perseverance. Most people who end up breaking their bad habits try and struggle repeatedly before they get it to work. You may not have instant success, but that doesn't mean you can't have it at all.

Chapter 2: QUESTIONING YOUR RELATIONSHIP WITH

ALCOHOL?

For many people, stopping drinking entails reaching "rock bottom" and seeking therapy through peer-support groups or in-person treatment institutions. At least, that's how many people used to think about alcoholism recovery. To re-evaluate if your connection with alcohol has a beneficial impact on your life, you don't have to lose everything or label yourself an "alcoholic" these days.

People are beginning to appreciate the benefits of abstaining from alcohol for some time, thanks to the recent popularity of 30-day challenges like Dry January and Sober October. However, if you're new to sober inquiry, you might not know where to start thinking about your drinking habits.

It does not have to be a daunting experience. You might think to yourself, "maybe I should get more sleep this week," or "maybe I should check in with myself about my alcohol use," just as you might think to yourself, "maybe I should check in with myself about my alcohol intake." Here's how to get started:

Ask yourself this question: Is alcohol still serving me?

Even if you don't see alcohol as a major issue in your life, Ruby Mehta, LCSW, director of clinical operations at Tempest, a digital recovery program, thinks it's a good idea to evaluate your relationship with alcohol from time to time.

"Ask yourself if alcohol is interfering with how you want to live or what you want to do. "Thinking about the effects of alcohol on the four key quadrants of your life can be helpful," Mehta suggests. These include the following:

•mental well-being

•physical well-being

•relationships

•work and daily routines

Consider what happens during and the day after drinking to see if alcohol has a detrimental impact on your health, relationships, work, school, or mental health.

•When you drink, do you get into more disputes with your friends and family?

•Is your hangover preventing you from taking advantage of a beautiful day outside?

•Is your productivity at work or school affected by how much you drank the night before?

According to Aimee Ellinwood, LPC, LAC, of Marisol Solarte-Erlacher, MA, LPC & Associates, "some signs that alcohol is having a negative impact on your life could include relationship turmoil, prolonged withdrawal, feeling out of control, drinking more to feel the same effects, and legal involvement related to alcohol use."

Consider what benefits alcohol provides to your life

According to Ellinwood, it's fine — and even common — to be unsure about changing your relationship with alcohol.

"A variety of approaches to managing alcohol consumption in social situations exist, including studying and practicing harm reduction strategies, managing moderation, and employing refusal skills. It's crucial to realize that you have the ability to make decisions," she adds.

When you consider the impact alcohol has on your life and determine that there are still some positives among the drawbacks, you've taken a crucial step toward understanding how your relationship with alcohol is working in general.

Mehta concurs. "It's vital to recognize that drinking alcohol may have certain benefits even if it's not serving you overall," she says. "It is vital to weigh the benefits and drawbacks of continuing to drink because it's ultimately up to you whether you want to attempt abstaining or reducing back."

Suppose you do decide to modify your relationship with alcohol. In that case, Mehta advises being "realistic about what you might have to give up to accomplish this change, at least at first."

If you can't picture socializing without having a drink in your hand, you're not alone. But, as Erin Stewart, MSW, points out, it gets easier over time.

"It will take time to adjust to a new normal," Stewart says, but practicing mindfulness (such as deep breathing) in social situations can help you focus on being completely present to the people you're speaking with.

She also suggests starting with an event where you're most at ease and relying on an alcohol-free beverage to help you adjust.

Think about the common risks of drinking alcohol

It's critical to educate yourself on the main risks of drinking if you're thinking about changing your relationship with alcohol.

According to Ellinwood, the following are some of the most common hazards associated with consuming alcohol:

•skewed judgment

•emotional vulnerability

•sleeping difficulties

•acting out of character

•putting one's own and others' safety in jeopardy

Furthermore, according to the Centers for Illness Control and Prevention (CDC)Trusted Source, heavy drinking increases your risk of:

•liver disease

•cancer

•heart disease

•high blood pressure

•stroke

Alcohol use is not only damaging to one's health, but "it can be particularly harmful to persons with depression, suicidal ideation, or anxiety because coming down from alcohol may exacerbate these symptoms," according to Mehta.

Take the first step

If you've considered it and want to try sobriety for a short time or for an indefinite period, getting started may be easier than you think.

"One of the wonderful aspects of COVID-19 this year is that sobriety support groups have gone virtual and are more easily accessible," Stewart explains. "I'd start by immersing yourself in a group, listening and sharing, and finding accountability companions or friends to help you get started with your new sober life. Lean on the

sober community for support. There's also Tempest, which provides a wealth of information for navigating sobriety."

Among the other programs are:

•The Alcoholics Anonymous (AA) group The Dharma of Recovery

•Smart Recovery

•Young People in Recovery

•In the Rooms

•LifeRing

•Celebrate Recovery

•Moderation Management

If groups aren't your thing, counseling is an excellent alternative.

"With substance use, it can sometimes become so habitual that we lose sight of our patterns of usage," Ellinwood says. "Recognizing our triggers for use and learning strategies to handle cravings and impulses can also be beneficial. Furthermore, the use of medication-assisted treatment (MAT) can greatly help people manage and reduce cravings."

Mehta also emphasizes the need to recognize if you were drinking to cope with something (for example, drinking in social settings owing to social anxiety) and finding other coping mechanisms for individuals seeking to quit drinking.

"Remember that alcohol was a coping strategy for you, and when it's gone, so is that coping mechanism," she says. "While this will be useful in the long run, it may be uncomfortable in the immediate term. Allowing yourself to try and discover what feels comfortable for you is something I would recommend."

Mehta suggests the following coping strategies:

•limiting social interactions to people you truly care about

•finding some good reads to indulge in (more on this later)

•starting a new hobby

•exercising

•meditation and breathwork

•finding calming scents

•beginning to work with a therapist or coach

"In general," she continues, "while your body and mind adjust to a life devoid of alcohol, I would advise you to be as gentle and compassionate with yourself as possible."

Build a network of support

When you start to reconsider your relationship with

alcohol, your friends and family may not be supportive, especially if they were the individuals with whom you used to drink.

Unfortunately, your new relationship with alcohol can make those same individuals feel condemned, which is why it's crucial to start by creating boundaries with the people in your life who still drink. In the end, it's your life and your choice, so "it's vital to think about creating boundaries, honoring your recovery goals, and prioritizing your needs," Ellinwood says.

In the early stages of sobriety, you can start setting boundaries by putting some distance between yourself and heavy drinkers and finding individuals who are in the same boat as you, adds Mehta.

Stewart recommends interacting with sober people on social media if you're having trouble finding support systems while trying to quit drinking or aren't sure how to establish sober friends.

"There are so many wonderful accounts and tiny tasks you can accomplish on social media. Annie Grace's challenges range in length from 30 days to a year. These are useful in detecting the effects of alcohol on the brain and how to rebuild our neural circuits with compassion for ourselves."

Explore resources and read some 'quit lit.'

Ellinwood recommends investigating and reading the Substance Abuse and Mental Health Services Administration website, which offers support and a 24/7 hotline if you

feel you have a more serious case of alcohol consumption (also recognized medically as alcohol use disorder).

However, if you're sober and inquisitive about your relationship with alcohol, as well as some of the effects it has on your body and mind, "stop lit" is a fantastic place to start.

This is a relatively new category of self-help literature that includes books written by people who have given up or drastically reduced alcohol consumption.

Recognize if you need professional help to quit

If you've tried and failed to cut back on alcohol, it's conceivable that you'll need professional assistance to help you stop drinking.

"If your attempts to reduce or eliminate your alcohol consumption have failed, it is critical to seek professional help," Ellinwood advises.

"It's also crucial to pay attention to what happens to your emotions when you stop drinking. If you've been using alcohol to cope with challenging or unpleasant emotions or experiences, they'll return immediately after you stop drinking. In these situations, it's critical to seek professional assistance to address and resolve the issues," she adds.

This is especially critical if you're having trouble quitting due to withdrawal symptoms, according to Stewart.

"If you are concerned that your body has become accustomed to this chemical, I will consult a doctor or a specialist (such as an addiction therapist)," she advises.

"Alcohol withdrawal is dangerous, and if you suspect you may be experiencing serious withdrawal symptoms,

I will consult a professional before attempting to quit drinking."

But how do you know whether you require professional assistance?

If you realize you need to drink progressively large amounts of alcohol to obtain the same effects you used to, or if you notice withdrawal symptoms such as:

•shakiness

•restlessness

•nausea

•excessive perspiration, Mehta recommends speaking with a healthcare practitioner.

It's worth contacting out even if you don't have these symptoms and just need extra support. "If you find yourself trying to stop repeatedly and failing, seeking professional

help from a therapist or an outpatient program may provide you with the best chance of long-term recovery," Mehta adds.

Above all, be gentle with yourself.

Although there is less stigma surrounding those on the spectrum of alcohol use disorder or even just sober inquisitive as compared to other substances, guilt surrounding alcohol and quitting drinking is still very real. In fact, after "lack of problem awareness," embarrassment was the second most common cause for people not seeking care, according to one study.

Traditional recovery programs focus on the label "alcoholic," which, although beneficial to those who like it, can feel stigmatizing to individuals suffering from problem drinking or those just beginning to explore sobriety.

It's crucial to realize that self-labeling isn't required to take a step back and reassess the role of alcohol in your life. As a result, Mehta advises being gentle with yourself and approaching this as an experiment.

"Keep in mind that stopping drinking can be difficult, so create reasonable goals for yourself," she advises. "Remember to congratulate yourself on tiny victories, such as your first night out without alcohol or informing a close friend about your intention to try sobriety or reduce your drinking."

Stewart also suggests that you find joy in sobriety by trying new things, moving your body, and scheduling alternate activities around your most likely drinking periods.

Chapter 3: I STOPPED DRINKING FOR 30 DAYS— HERE IS

WHAT IT DID TO MY MIND, BODY, AND SKIN

It was Memorial Day weekend. A close mate, Victoria, and I had jetted up to Santa Barbara to celebrate the start of summer for a day of wine tasting. We had spent the day strolling from winery to winery, tasting a variety of pinots, both red and white, and both of us were sporting a festive buzz on our last day of tasting. It was more of a goodbye party because I'd embark on a sober 30 days starting June 1.

I almost couldn't believe it, but I didn't give myself so much as a sip of a friend's rosé for the entire month of June. I know it doesn't sound like a big deal for some people to go 30 days without alcohol, but I'd never done it before. I hadn't gone more than a dry week since high school when I thought about it. Alcohol was already playing a relatively present part of my life at 24. I wasn't drunk as I was in college (my gut-wrenching hangovers wouldn't encourage that).

Yet alcohol was always closely tied up with my life. As

an experiment, I wanted to see just how, without it, I could work.

Victoria and I were going out to the outdoor patio of the winery to finish our final glass when we stumbled (quite literally) across a chalkboard sign that read, "No wine past this point." I stood at the front steps and drank my last drink, and we took a ride from Lyft. The next day I will wake up a sober woman.

Why I Quit Drinking?

I want to dig a little further into why I wanted to go booze-free before getting into my 30-day experiment. First of all, I was willing to ease some of alcohol's harmful effects that I still bear.

For starters, I would have started eating a plant-based diet about six months before, and a lot of the vegan community is sober as well. It goes hand in hand with a mentality that is clean-eating. The vegans I know who don't drink seem extraordinarily vibrant and healthy, and I was curious to see if alcohol giving up would do the same for me.

I was also inspired by tales from friends who had gone without drinking long stretches before. My boyfriend has spent 30 days refusing alcohol, and the results have been nothing short of spectacular. He lost weight, his eczema and rosacea subsided, and in the end, he appeared a happier, more successful individual overall. He told me the first

week was tough, but you don't even miss the alcohol anymore after that. You don't even know why you liked this.

And because it all appealed to me, eating less, feeling brighter, and having healthy skin, I knew I was all-in to give this a shot.

Benefits of Quitting Alcohol

Higher energy levels

Better quality of sleep

Improved skin health and hydration

According to registered dietitian Jenny Champion, sugar cravings, excess calorie consumption, dehydrated skin, fuzzy concentration, and bad moods can be caused by just casual drinking. Not only does alcohol produce almost twice as many calories as vegetables, but blended drinks are also full of sugar fruit juice — so you're missing something if you watch your diet but don't work out at night. But alcohol doesn't only trigger sugar cravings; it flat out makes you crave food. Cravings and lowered inhibitions that come with alcohol are perfect for drinks loaded with carbs and sugar but not perfect for feeling better.

Not only does alcohol contain twice as many calories as carbohydrates, but mixed drinks are often full of sugary fruit juice.

.

Thinking of the next morning, who among us got drunk and forgot to take off our makeup or forget our skincare routine in favor of a makeup wipe? Just being unwavering with skincare benefits the skin. It's well known, however, that alcohol itself has adverse effects on your skin. A by-product of alcohol metabolization is acetaldehyde, which not only dehydrates your body but also your skin. Unfortunately, no amount of water you drink can do away with this particular negative effect; the best you can expect to do is to dilute it. Booze also dilates your pores and acts as an inflammatory, releasing histamine, which is why your skin gets so red and blotchy and stays so bad a few days later.

Finally, when I thought deeply about it, it just seemed odd to me that something as easy as a drink could have such life-changing and mind-altering effects on people. It seems that alcohol has set this spell upon us. For so many reasons, we empty our glasses: as

payment, as a medicine, as social lubrication, as an escape. When there's something positive going on, we drink. When we drink, something bad happens. Sometimes we drink for no reason at all. I've decided that I no longer wanted to be under that influence.

What to Expect

It has to be stated: My sober month has been tough. I

was most excited at the beginning to see the positive effects it would have on my skin. That might be irrational, but I wanted to observe major improvements immediately: a brightened skin, a dewier finish, and fewer blemishes. When nothing, a week into the challenge seemed different, I started questioning why I did it in the first place.

Going an alcohol-free month also teaches you about the drinking habit. This is important information if you want to try to cut back on alcohol in the future again. I often drink three to four nights a week, but when I do, I prefer only to have one or two glasses.

When I go past two glasses on those occasions, alcohol starts to be a problem for me.

To be honest, it's hard to tell whether or not the huge blemish on my cheek before I started drinking was linked to alcohol. I've recently had a skin problem that rivaled the one at the end of my sober month. A beautician later told me my imperfections probably had more to do with hormones and stress than anything else. I know, a little bit anti-climactic. But that rough, pinkish patch of skin right next to my eye was certainly alcohol-related. It was a nasty spot of eczema, which I had been fighting for nearly a year. My eczema is not painful or itching; it's just unsightly. The scaly texture is such that I can't hide it with makeup, and even prescription steroid creams couldn't make it go away. To date, the only treatment that has worked to clear my eczema is giving up alcohol. About two weeks in, for the first time in months, the inflamed, crinkled skin softens. Certified nutritionist Dana James suggests that a reaction to yeast may be causing my eczema. "You've lowered your contact with it by taking the alcohol out and reducing the symptoms," she told me.

A by-product of alcohol metabolization is acetaldehyde, which not only dehydrates your body but your skin too.

Although at the end of the month, my eczema re-emerged slightly, that initial disappearing act was substantial. I also found that the parts of my face, which tended to get flaky looked a little more hydrated by week two of my experiment.

Actually, for the last two weeks of my sober month, my

skin quality appeared to remain relatively constant. Yet after the 30 days had finished and I started to drink again, it quickly returned to its unhealthy state. To put it plainly, there is no questioning the influence of alcohol on our skin—you just have to be aware to see that.

Side Effects

I'm going to say something that could upset you but not even as much as it disappointed me: I gained weight during my month without alcohol —around 3 pounds, to be exact. I think the main reason is that during those 30 days, I found myself eating out in restaurants a lot — three or four nights a week, indulging in rich Thai curries and oily plates of pasta. I convinced myself that I was saving so many calories that I could eat pretty much anything I wanted by not drinking. The reasoning hasn't served me well. Of course, the meals were plant-based and followed by sparkling water instead of wine, but it was enough to tip the scale to eat those large portions of restaurant food. (As a reminder, I don't personally own a scale and rarely weigh myself; I did so purely for this experiment's sake.) Speaking of dining out, it did not seem like my social life was suffering from my sobriety, as I was concerned. We simply decided to grab a bite to eat instead of a drink at a bar when making plans with friends. (This also led to my heightened consumption of restaurant calories.)

Each time I got home at a respectable hour, never woke up hungover, and everybody was always having fun. Waking up feeling healthy and well-rested every day has been one of my favorite aspects of not drinking for a month. As I have said, these days, I seldom get drunk enough to cause crippling hangovers. Yet, at times, two drinks are all that's needed to make me feel foggy and bloated the next day. I didn't get up earlier than usual, but I certainly squeezed in an extra half hour every night. Winding down with a drink after work always inspired me to go to bed before. This had to do more with the boredom—10 p.m. Will roll around and joyful buzz without any kind of light

The Final Takeaway

I'd be lying if I said I wasn't disappointed that after 30 days without drinking, there were no more drastic changes to my body. All the experiences of friends of mine

seemed so much more worthwhile. I believe the reason for this has to do with another unexpected but important lesson that I learned from this experiment.

A fading eczema patch and an additional 30 minutes of sleep are no doubt useful rewards. But the most remarkable thing I've learned from my alcohol-free 30 days — the thing that made it all worth doing — is that it taught me exactly what function alcohol serves in my life.

During the month, there were two occasions when I missed the most alcohol. The first came at the end of a hard workday after coming in the door when all I wanted was to put my feet up and have a glass of wine. The other was when I was in a big group during social outings, and everyone else was drinking but me. For different purposes, everybody uses alcohol, and obviously, these are mine: I use alcohol as a small, private reward for myself and as a way of bonding in large social settings. When something frustrating or bad happened, I didn't crave a cocktail. When I felt anxious and wanted to relax, I didn't miss it on a date night with my boyfriend or during awkward social circumstances. These are not the roles played by alcohol in my life. So, I'm really curious to know that.

So, I've put myself on a strict two-drink maximum since my 30-day experiment. Given my drinking habits, this has become a much better way for me to make sure I'm drinking in moderation.

After all, it's possible to lead a healthy lifestyle as a moderate drinker, according to experts (as long as you don't struggle with an addiction or drinking problem, that is). "If you're living an active and balanced lifestyle that involves a diet rich in nutrients, the occasional drink shouldn't be a concern," promises John Ford, a Find Your Trainer personal trainer. The trick is to determine what function alcohol is serving in your life and fix any harmful behaviors. That's just what helped me for a month, going sober.

In the end, I didn't lose ten years off my face or 10 pounds off my body through my 30 days without alcohol. But it enabled me to learn more about my personality, my conduct, and my health. For me, that's something worth clinking a glass to.

Chapter 4: ALCOHOL WITHDRAWAL SYMPTOMS

What Is Alcohol Withdrawal?

When you drink alcohol regularly for weeks, months, or years when you quit or severely cut down on how much you drink, you might have both mental and physical issues. This is termed withdrawal from alcohol. Symptoms may be mild to severe.

When you drink just once and then you stop, it is unlikely you will have signs of withdrawal. However, if you have been through alcohol withdrawal once, you are more likely to go through it again the next time you call it quits.

What Causes It?

Alcohol has what physicians call a depressive effect on the system. It slows the functioning of the brain and changes the way your nerves send out messages.

Over time, the central nervous system adjusts to still having alcohol around every time. The body is working hard to keep the brain alert and keep the nerves communicating with each other.

When the level of alcohol abruptly decreases, the brain

stays in that keyed-up state. That is what triggers withdrawal.

What Are the Symptoms?

They can vary from mild to serious. What happens depends on how much and how long you've been drinking alcohol.

Generally, the mild signs start as early as 6 hours after you put down your bottle. Can include:

Headache

Shaky hands

Anxiety

Nausea

Insomnia

Vomiting

Sweating

More serious problems range from 12 to 24-hour hallucinations after the last drink to seizures within the first two days after you stop. You can see, feel or hear stuff that doesn't exist.

That's not the same as delirium tremens or DTs. DTs typically start 48 to 72 hours after you put the glass down. Such symptoms include intense visions and delusions. Only about 5 percent of people with withdrawal from alcohol have them. Those that do may also have:

Racing heart

Confusion

High blood pressure

Heavy sweating

Fever

How Is Withdrawal Diagnosed?

When the doctor suspects you might have withdrawn, he'll ask you questions about your history of drinking and whether you've stopped recently. He will want to know if you have ever experienced withdrawal before.

He'll talk about your symptoms too. He'll be checking for any medical problems during an assessment to see whether they may be to blame.

Treatment

Your doctor will direct you about the type of care you need. If you have a serious health problem or have had extreme withdrawals in the past, you would generally need little more than a supportive atmosphere to get you through it; this includes:

Soft lighting

A quiet place

Healthy food and lots of fluids

A positive, supportive atmosphere

Limited contact with people

When your blood pressure, pulse, or body temperature increases, or if you have more serious symptoms such as seizures and hallucinations, seek urgent medical attention (dial 911). Your doctor may prescribe medication for the inpatient and medications.

Popular medications include benzodiazepines that help relieve symptoms such as anxiety, insomnia, and seizures. Along with other medications, you can even take anti- seizure medicines and antipsychotics.

Can You Prevent It?

Treating withdrawal of alcohol is a short-term remedy that does not solve the core problem. When discussing pain relief with your doctor, seeking treatment for substance abuse or dependency is a smart idea. You can get advice from the doctor to help you avoid drinking.

Chapter 5: ALCOHOL WITHDRAWAL SYNDROME

The scope of alcohol withdrawal symptoms varies from mild symptoms such as fatigue and tremulousness to serious problems such as hallucinations during withdrawal and delirium tremens. While the history and physical examination are typically adequate to diagnose alcohol withdrawal syndrome, there may be similar signs in other circumstances. Most patients with withdrawal from alcohol can be treated as outpatients safely and effectively. Pharmacological interventions include the use of alcohol-responsive drugs. Benzodiazepines, the agents of choice, can be administered on a set schedule or caused by symptoms. Carbamazepine is a safe alternative to a benzodiazepine in ambulatory care of patients with mild to moderate symptoms of withdrawal from alcohol. Drugs such as haloperidol, beta-blockers, clonidine, and phenytoin can be used to treat withdrawal symptoms as adjuncts to benzodiazepine. Alcohol detox therapy should be followed by alcohol dependency therapy.

In 1992, 13.8 million Americans met the alcohol abuse or dependence criteria specified in the Mental Disorders

Diagnostic and Statistical Manual, Fourth Edition, Text Review (DSM-IV-TR). In 2000, 226,000 patients were discharged from short-stay hospitals (excluding Veteran Affairs and other federal hospitals). So, up to 2 million Americans may experience symptoms of alcohol withdrawal every year.

Pathophysiology

Several mechanisms mediate drug withdrawal syndrome. The brain maintains neurochemical equilibrium by neurotransmitters which are inhibitory and excitatory. The major neurotransmitter inhibitory is π-aminobutyric acid (GABA), which works with GABA-alpha (GABA-A)

One of the biggest exciting neurotransmitters is glutamate which acts through the neuroreceptor of N-methyl-D-aspartate (NMDA).

Alcohol increases GABA's effect on GABA-A neuroreceptors, resulting in reduced overall excitability throughout the brain. Chronic alcohol consumption results in a compensatory reduction in GABA-A neuroreceptor response to GABA, as shown by the increasing tolerance of alcohol impact.

Alcohol activates the neuroreceptors of NMDA, and prolonged exposure to alcohol results in these receptors being regulated upwards. Abrupt cessation of exposure to alcohol results in brain hyperexcitability, as alcohol-inhibited receptors are no longer inhibited. Hyperexcitability of the brain clinically expresses itself as fear, irritability,

agitation, and tremors. Extreme symptoms include hallucinations with alcohol withdrawal and tremors with delirium.

The "kindling" effect is an important concept in both alcohol dependence and alcohol withdrawal; the term refers to the long-lasting changes in neurons following repeated detoxification. Recurrent detoxification is postulated to increase addictive thoughts or the craving for alcohol. Kindling describes the finding that subsequent periods of alcohol withdrawal appear to intensify slowly.

While the importance of kindling in the withdrawal of alcohol is being debated, this phenomenon may be significant in selecting drugs for withdrawal care. When certain medicines decrease the enhanced effect, they may become favored agents.

Withdrawal Symptoms

Table 2 lists the continuum of withdrawal symptoms and the period for these symptoms to occur following cessation of alcohol use. Alcohol withdrawal symptoms typically apply proportionately to the amount of drug intake and the duration of a patient's recent pattern of drinking. Most patients in any episode of alcohol withdrawal have a broad set of symptoms.

There can be mild withdrawal effects when the patient still has a detectable amount of alcohol in the blood. These symptoms may include sleeplessness, mild anxiety, and tremor. Alcoholic hallucinosis patients experience visual, auditory, or tactile hallucinations but otherwise have strong sensory faculties.

Withdrawal seizures are more common in patients with a history of repeated detoxifying episodes. Whether seizures are focal, if there is no clear history of recent abstinence from drinking, seizures occur more than 48 hours after the patient's last drink, or whether the patient has a history of fever or injuries, factors other than alcohol withdrawal should be considered.

The delirium of alcohol withdrawal, or delirium tremens, is characterized by the clouding of consciousness and hallucinations. Delirium tremor episodes have a mortality rate of 1 to 5 percent. Risk factors for the development of alcohol withdrawal include concurrent acute medical illness, daily heavy alcohol consumption, history of delirium tremens or older age, withdrawal seizures, abnormal liver function, and more severe withdrawal symptoms on presentation.

Evaluation of the Patient in Alcohol Withdrawal

History and physical exam determine the diagnosis and extent of withdrawal from alcohol. Important historical details include the quantity of alcoholic intake, length of alcohol consumption, the period since last drink, past withdrawals of alcohol, the existence of related medical or psychiatric problems, and abuse of other agents. The physical examination will determine, in addition to detecting withdrawal symptoms, potential complicating medical problems, including arrhythmias, congestive heart failure, coronary artery disease, gastrointestinal bleeding, allergies, liver disease, weakness of the nervous system, and pancreatitis. Basic lab examinations include a full blood count, liver function checks, urine drug examination, and blood alcohol and electrolyte level determination.

The revised scale of the Clinical Institute Withdrawal Assessment for Alcohol (CIWA- Ar) is a validated 10-point evaluation tool that can measure the severity of alcohol withdrawal syndrome and track and treat patient's withdrawal (Figure 1). CIWA-Ar scores of 8 points or less correspond to mild withdrawal, and 9 to 15 points correspond to severe withdrawal. The clinical image should be considered when using the CIWA- Ar since medical and psychological problems can resemble alcohol withdrawal symptoms. Additionally, certain medicines (e.g., beta-blockers) may moderate these symptoms.

Differential Diagnosis

Alcohol withdrawal syndrome and other conditions may be confused. Thyrotoxicosis, anticholinergic drug overdose, and the use of amphetamine or cocaine may lead to symptoms of increased sympathetic activity and mental changes. Infection or illness of the central nervous system may cause hallucinations and changes in mental status.

Removal from other sedative-hypnotic agents induces symptoms similar to those that occur in the condition of withdrawal from alcohol.

Goals of Treatment

The American Society of Addiction Medicine specifies

three specific aims for the detoxification of alcohol and other substances: (1) "providing a healthy removal from the drug(s) of dependency and enabling the patient to become drug-free;" (2) "providing a compassionate removal and thereby maintaining the integrity of the

patient;" and (3) "preparing the patient for the continued treatment of his or her dependency on the medication."

General Care

Any blood gas, electrolytes, or nutritional irregularities should be corrected. In patients with extreme withdrawal may require intravenous fluids due to excessive loss of fluid through hyperthermia, sweating, and vomiting. Intravenous fluids in patients with less serious withdrawal should not be regularly administered, as these patients may become overhydrated.

It has not been shown to improve withdrawal symptoms through regular administration of magnesium sulfate, but supplementation is necessary if a patient is in hypomagnesemia. During alcohol detox therapy, multivitamins and thiamine (100 mg per day) should be given. If intravenous fluids are administered, thiamine (100 mg intravenously) should be given before glucose is released to prevent Wernicke's encephalopathy from developing.

Medication Regimens

Drugs can be administered using fixed-schedule or symptom-triggered regimens (Table 3). Benzodiazepine doses are administered at regular intervals with a fixed-schedule regimen, and additional doses of the drug are administered as required depending on the severity of the withdrawal symptoms. Medication is offered in a symptom-triggered regime only if the CIWA-Ar score is greater than 8 points.

Symptom-triggered regimes have been shown to result in less overall medication administration and provide a shorter treatment period. In one randomized, double-blind clinical trial,11 patients in the symptom-triggered group received an average of 100 mg of chlordiazepoxide. In contrast, patients in the fixed-schedule group received an average of 425 mg. The mean treatment period in the symptom-triggered group was nine hours, compared with 68 hours in the fixed-schedule group. Patients were removed from the study if they had underlying medical or mental disorders from any cause that involved hospitalization or seizure

Another trial yielded similar findings, with patients receiving an average of 231.4 mg of oxazepam in the fixed-schedule group and those receiving 37.5 mg in the symptom- triggered group. For the patients in the group affected by the symptoms, 61 percent got

no oxazepam. The study excluded people with severe psychological, emotional, or medical comorbidities.

The use of symptom-triggered therapy will require clinical staff training. If this instruction has not been provided, pharmacotherapy should be used on a set schedule.

Choice of Treatment Setting

Outpatient detoxification is safe and successful in most patients with mild to moderate withdrawal symptoms and costs less than inpatient care. However, certain patients should be considered for inpatient treatment irrespective of the severity of their symptoms. Indicative signs for inpatient alcohol detoxification are as follows: serious withdrawal symptoms, history of withdrawal seizures or delirium tremors, numerous prior detoxifications, concomitant mental or medical disorder, recent high alcohol intake rates, pregnancy, and lack of a stable support network.

When ambulatory treatment is preferred, the patient should be reviewed regularly. The patient and support person(s) should be advised on how to administer the withdrawal drug, the side effects of the drug, the possible symptoms of withdrawal, and what to do if symptoms worsen. Small amounts of withdrawal medication should be administered during each visit; thiamine and multivitamins should also be administered. Due to the lack of close supervision in outpatient care, a set schedule regime should be used.

PHARMACOLOGICAL TREATMENT OF WITHDRAWAL

Benzodiazepines

Pharmacological diagnosis of alcohol withdrawal syndrome includes the use of drugs that do not interact. Benzodiazepines are safe and effective, particularly in preventing or treating seizures and delirium, and are the preferred agents for treating alcohol withdrawal syndrome symptoms.

The physician's choice is dependent on the pharmacokinetics. Diazepam (Valium) and chlordiazepoxide (Librium) are long-acting drugs that have proven effective in treating symptoms of alcohol withdrawal. Withdrawal is quicker because of the long half-life of these drugs, and signs of rebound withdrawal are less likely to occur. Lorazepam (Ativan) and oxazepam (Serax) function immediately and have outstanding efficacy records. Treatment with these agents, particularly the elderly and those with liver

failure, may be preferable in patients who metabolize medications less effective. Lorazepam is the only benzodiazepine whose intramuscular absorption is predictable (if intramuscular administration is necessary).

Rarely, extremely high dosages of benzodiazepines are needed to control the symptoms of withdrawal from alcohol. Dosages of diazepam as high as 2,000 mg a day were administered. Since physicians are often hesitant to prescribe extremely high dosages, undertreatment of alcohol withdrawal is a common issue.

One randomized controlled trial (RCT)19 confirmed previous findings that carbamazepine in patients with mild to moderate symptoms is an important alternative to benzodiazepines in treating alcohol withdrawal syndrome. Patients in the study received 800 mg of carbamazepine on day one, with the dosage tapered to 200 mg by day five. Carbamazepine (Tegretol) also tends to relieve drug cravings following withdrawal. It is not sedating and has little abuse potential. While carbamazepine is commonly used in Europe, its use in the United States has been restricted by inadequate evidence that it prevents seizures and delirium.

ADJUNCTIVE AGENTS

In the diagnosis of alcohol withdrawal syndrome, some drugs can be effective adjuncts to benzodiazepines. These drugs should not, however, be used as monotherapy.

Haloperidol (Haldol) can treat anxiety and hallucinations, and it can decrease the risk of seizures. The use of atenolol (Tenormin) in combination with oxazepam has been shown to improve symptoms faster and more effectively alleviate drug cravings than oxazepam alone.

Adjunctive treatment with a beta-blocker should be considered in patients with coronary artery disease who may not tolerate the strain on the cardiovascular system that alcohol withdrawal can impose. Clonidine (Catapres) has also been shown to enhance autonomic withdrawal symptoms. While phenytoin (Dilantin) does not treat withdrawal seizures, it is an appropriate alternative in patients with an underlying seizure disorder.

Patient Follow-Up

Alcohol withdrawal syndrome therapy should be accompanied by alcohol dependency therapy. Withdrawal therapy alone does not resolve the underlying addiction disorder, providing no hope for long-term abstinence.

Brief interventions in patients with alcohol dependency are helpful in the outpatient setting, but more intensive treatments can be needed in patients with alcohol dependence. It has been shown that anticonvulsant topiramate (Topamax) is an important adjunctive drug for reducing alcohol intake and abstinence in alcohol-dependent patients

After attending 12-step programs like Alcoholics Anonymous and Narcotics Anonymous, some patients produce positive results. Many patients benefit from stays in comprehensive treatment facilities, including a 12-step model, cognitive-behavioral therapy, and family therapy. Alcohol withdrawal syndrome therapy should complement an individualized, intensive treatment plan, or at least as many components of a plan as the patient can handle and afford.

Future Directions

Some drugs showed early promise in treating withdrawal from alcohol. A single 10-mg dose of baclofen in one case report involving five patients relieved severe withdrawal symptoms. In a preliminary RCT, baclofen also minimized cravings in patients addicted to alcohol.

In small trials, gabapentin, which is structurally similar to GABA, successfully treated alcohol withdrawal. The low toxicity of gabapentin makes it a promising agent. In another study, the vigabatrin anticonvulsant agent, which blocks GABA transaminase irreversibly, diminished withdrawal symptoms after three days of treatment.

Prevention

Early identification of problem drinking allows complications to be prevented or treated, including severe withdrawal. The U.S. Preventive Services Task Force recommends screening patients through a careful history or standardized screening questionnaire for problematic drinking. Patients undergoing preoperative assessment should also be screened because the cessation of alcohol will hinder recovery from surgery. Elective surgery should be delayed until the addicted patient has had no alcohol for 7 to 10 days.

Chapter 6: WAYS TO CURB YOUR DRINKING

Do you have any concerns regarding your alcohol consumption? Perhaps you think you're drinking too much or too frequently. Perhaps it's a bad habit you'd like to break.

It's usually a good idea to check with your doctor first; she should be able to advise you on whether you should cut back or abstain. People addicted to alcohol or who have other medical or mental health issues should abstain from drinking entirely.

However, many people may gain simply by reducing their spending. If your doctor advises you to cut back on your alcohol consumption, the National Institute on Alcohol Abuse and Alcoholism (NIAAA) suggests the following steps:

1.Put it down on paper. Making a list of reasons to stop drinking, such as feeling better, sleeping better, or enhancing your relationships, might help you stay motivated.

2.Make a drinking target for yourself. Set a limit on the amount of alcohol you will consume. Drinking should be limited to one standard drink per day for women and men 65 and older and two standard drinks per day for men younger than 65. For those with specific medical issues or for some elderly adults, these limitations may be too high. Your doctor can assist you in deciding what is best for you.

3.Keep track of your drinking in a journal. Keep track of every drink you have for three to four weeks. Include details on what you drank, how much you drank, and where you were. When you compare this to your goal, you'll see how far you've come. Talk to your doctor or another health expert if you're having problems keeping to your goal.

4.Don't store alcoholic beverages in your home. If you don't have any alcohol at home, you'll be able to cut down on your drinking.

5.Sip slowly. Sip your beverage. After you've had an alcoholic beverage, drink some soda, water, or juice. Never consume alcohol on an empty stomach.

6.Schedule no-alcohol days. Make a weekly decision to skip a day or two of drinking. You might want to try going without alcohol for a week or a month to see how you feel physically and mentally. Taking a vacation from alcohol can help you cut down on your drinking.

7.Keep an eye out for peer pressure. Practice respectfully saying no. You are not forced to drink just because others are, and you should not take every drink handed to you. People that encourage you to drink should be avoided.

8.Keep yourself occupied. Take a walk, participate in sports, eat out, or see a movie. Pick up a new activity or return to an old one when you're at home. Painting, playing board games, learning a musical instrument, and woodworking is excellent alternatives to drinking.

9.Seek assistance. It's not always easy to cut back on your drinking. Make it clear to your friends and family that you require their assistance. A doctor, counselor, or therapist may be able to assist you.

10.Avoid succumbing to temptation. Avoid people and settings that make you feel compelled to drink. If you associate drinking with certain occasions, such as holidays or vacations, make a strategy for dealing with them ahead of time. Keep an eye on your emotions. You may be tempted to reach for a drink when you're anxious, lonely, or furious. Attempt to develop new, healthy stress coping mechanisms.

11.Don't give up. The majority of persons who successfully reduce or stop drinking do so after multiple efforts. Setbacks are inevitable, but don't let them deter you from achieving your long-term goal. Because the process normally necessitates continual work, there is no definitive endpoint.

Some of these tactics, such as avoiding peer pressure, staying busy, asking for help, being aware of temptation, and persevering, can also benefit persons who want to abstain entirely from alcohol.

TIPS TO HELP YOU STOP DRINKING ALCOHOL

1.Start with a plan.

Before you begin, sit down and explore your alternatives. Select a framework that works for you and consider the finer points. What will you do if you have a strong desire to drink? If you require assistance, who will you contact? Prepare some coping tactics ahead of time and be ready to implement them.

It's also beneficial to be aware of your drinking habits and triggers. Plan ahead of time to avoid situations that attract you to drink, and be prepared to distract yourself if alcohol does occur. Overall, the better you know yourself and the more you prepare, the more resilient you will be when things get tough.

2.Establish a strong support group

With friends, allies, coaches, or all of the above, quitting is considerably easier. One approach to locate a supportive community is to join groups like Alcoholics Anonymous 1 (AA) or alternatives like SMART recovery2. A sponsor or a rehabilitation coach may also be beneficial. This entails having a knowledgeable ally who can keep you on track, provide sound counsel, and hold you accountable when necessary.

Finally, merely informing friends and family about your

plans and soliciting their support can go a long way. There will be fewer drinking triggers if people are aware of your situation and willing to assist you. When things get tough, you'll have somebody to talk to.

3.Think about medication as a possibility.

Although alcohol addiction medication is not as well-known as AA or treatment, it is one of the most successful methods for quitting drinking. The Sinclair Method, for example, has shown that taking naltrexone to curb alcohol cravings has a 78 percent long-term success rate.

The FDA has approved three drugs for the treatment of alcoholism: naltrexone, acamprosate, and disulfiram. Gabapentin, baclofen, and topiramate are just a few of the medications that are prescribed off-label. Each of these methods works differently, but they can help you overcome your physical alcohol dependence. This can make the mental battle a lot simpler.

4.Consult your physician before going cold turkey.

This is a crucial point: Alcohol withdrawal can be harmful, even lethal, in some situations. This may not be the case for you, but following a doctor's advice can help you stay safe. Medical counseling can also introduce you to beneficial resources suitable for your condition, even if you don't foresee severe withdrawal symptoms.

5.Start with a moderate or cutback approach.

It is typically simpler to quit drinking altogether if you reduce your drinking beforehand. Moderation can be difficult to accomplish, but there are a variety of tactics that might assist. The National Institute on Alcohol Abuse and Alcoholism has some excellent suggestions for reducing alcohol consumption. 3. Medications such as naltrexone can also help a lot.

One advantage of cutting back ahead of time is that withdrawal symptoms are less intense. Moderation may also prove to be a beneficial long-term approach for you. Although conventional wisdom implies that abstinence is the sole option, many people

find that moderation is possible. The greatest course to choose is usually the one that is most effective for you.

6.Practice Self-Care Techniques

Some folks start incorporating a long stroll into their daily routine. Some people begin meditating. Before going to bed, some people recite positive affirmations. Whatever method works best for you, attempt to develop a set of routines that will help you maintain a sense of balance and mindfulness.

It's difficult to break a long-standing habit. There will be good days and bad days. It's best to prepare for it and have some strategies in place. Although chatting to a buddy or a coach can help, it's equally important to consider what you do on your own time. Be gentle to yourself, keep a cheerful attitude, and prepare some self-care measures.

This leads us to the next point:

7.Find new ways to replace alcohol in your life.

Consider going to the gym after work instead of drinking a beer. Look for social groups that share common interests, such as music, sports, arts and crafts, or hiking. Fill your schedule with activities that you can do instead of drinking, and watch as they gradually take over your life.

You might be amazed at how many social chances are available without booze. The sober inquisitive movement has increased alcohol-free nightlife. There are also applications and online communities 4 that can help you connect with other sober people who share your interests.

In the near term, new interests and pursuits that do not include drinking alcohol will distract you. They'll naturally guide you toward a more fulfilling, alcohol-free personal life as time goes on.

8.Set long-term goals.

Begin by making a list of the reasons you wish to cut back or quit. Maybe you want to be a better parent, or you want to feel healthier, or you want to improve your job performance. Write these goals down and keep them with you as a reminder when you first stop drinking. Then, as you grow, reward yourself. If it's been a month since you've had a drink, treat yourself to a good meal or a new outfit. To move forward, use positive reinforcement and big-picture thinking.

This can be challenging at first. However, as more positive improvements occur, it will become simpler. Seeing tangible evidence that you are getting healthier or improving your family life is a great drive to stay away from alcohol. Knowing that your early aims contributed to your success demonstrates your strength and determination.

9.Never Give Up

For many people, quitting alcohol is a hard process with numerous setbacks. Allowing oneself to be disheartened is a mistake. Many others who had succeeded before you had difficult obstacles along the way, and it took them multiple tries to figure out what worked best for them.

What matters is that you keep going. If one option fails, start over and try another. There are many different programs, techniques, and approaches for quitting drinking. One of them is almost certainly going to work for you. If the procedure takes a long time, keep in mind that you are making a significant change in your life and health.

Large-scale changes require time. That's one of the reasons why it can feel so good when you finally succeed.

Chapter 7: PLANNING FOR ALCOHOL OR DRUG RELAPSE

When you want to avoid using alcohol or narcotics, you should take steps to stay drug- free or sober. It's very hard to stop using substances, whether it's alcohol or drugs you're using. The first time they try, very few people succeed. There is likely to be a break or a relapse.

•A drop is the first time you use the substance or drink again after stopping or short periods of later use.

•A relapse can't stay drug-free or drug-sober over time. It can occur if you have a series of near lapses or a lapse over a longer period leading to the heavier use of drugs or alcohol. It most often occurs a couple of months after you stop using drugs or alcohol.

If there's a slipup or relapse, that may mean you've just messed up. If that's valid for you, then accept the error and move on. Start finding out why you've relapsed and made changes in your life so it won't happen again. You may even need additional medical treatment or more time for support programs like Narcotics Anonymous, LifeRing, or Alcoholics Anonymous.

You may have many relapses, whether you have managed to avoid using the drug on your own or sought support. Relapses typically occur less often as time goes by and are shorter.

Have a relapse plan

Consider you may be getting a relapse. This might be easier to deal with if you think about what to do with a relapse before it happens.

Speak to support experts on what to do if you have a relapse. Such individuals can include your sponsor or doctor, psychologist, family, colleagues, and community support. Decide who to call, where to go, and what to do if a question occurs. There are people you should turn to, including your sponsor, your psychiatrist, your psychologist, or a hotline for the crisis.

Think about your triggers

Triggers are things that might cause you to have a relapse. They may include:

•Certain people. Running into people with whom you drank or used drugs can cause memories and a desire to use drugs or alcohol again. They might encourage you to use drugs or alcohol if you meet these people.

•Certain places. Walking into a bar, a friend's home, or a park where you have been drinking or using drugs can cause a craving. Even being in the same area may cause some cravings.

•Certain things. You can connect objects to alcohol or drug use. Finding a syringe or crack pipe, for example, might cause memories.

•Certain times. A craving may happen on certain days or times of the day, holidays, or weather. That depends on the drug or alcohol experiences.

•Certain smells, sounds, and sensations. A cause may be the scent of the drug, a cigarette, or a meal. It may also trigger a longing for a rainy day, an album, or a TV program.

•Stress. Stress is a definite catalyst. Any situation in which you feel stress increases your chance of a relapse.

•Certain situations. Social events, parties, or being alone may make you think about taking a drink or trying drugs.

Writing down the causes and learning about them will help. Are any more likely than others to cause a relapse? Rank the causes most likely to cause a relapse to the least likely to cause a relapse.

Decide on how to handle your triggers. You need to avoid certain circumstances or individuals or stay away from a favorite activity or location. When you know that you can't stop a cause, bring in a friend to help you.

If you lapse or relapse

•Avoid drinking alcohol at once or taking the drug. Get rid of this thing. Leave where you are in the situation.

•Rest assured. Remember, you have a strategy, and remember how hard you've worked to stay drug-free or sober.

•Get help immediately. Call the people listed in your

plan, or go to the locations specified in your plan.

•Focus on what happened after you started drinking alcohol or taking drugs. Find out what caused you to relapse and how to stop it happening again. Place that in your strategy.

Chapter 8: WHAT HAPPENS TO YOUR BODY WHEN YOU

STOP DRINKING ALCOHOL

You might be able to avoid accidents.

At least half of all catastrophic trauma injuries and deaths, such as burns, drownings, and killings, are caused by alcohol. It's also involved in four out of every ten fatal falls, road accidents, and suicides. To be safe, you don't have to go fully dry. Even a third reduction in drinking can reduce the number of injuries and sick days.

Your Heart Is Getting Better

You may believe that drinking a glass of red wine or other alcoholic beverages regularly is good for your heart. However, this may not be true, or may just be true for mild drinkers (less than one drink a day). If you use more than that, cutting back or quitting may help lower your blood pressure, triglyceride levels, and heart failure risk.

It's Possible That Your Liver Will Heal

Toxins are filtered by your liver. Alcohol is also harmful to your cells. Heavy drinking

— at least 15 drinks per week for males and eight drinks per week for women — can harm the liver and lead to fatty liver, cirrhosis, and other complications. The good news is that your liver can mend and even renew itself. As a result, drinking less or quitting is always a good idea.

You Might Lose Weight

A glass of ordinary beer contains approximately 150 calories, while a serving of wine contains approximately 120 calories. Alcohol increases your hunger on top of those essentially empty calories. It also makes you more impulsive, allowing you to succumb to the fries and other menu temptations. As a result, if you refrain from drinking alcohol, the number on your scale may begin to decrease.

It's possible that your relationships will improve.

Socially consumed alcohol in moderation can improve your mood and help you bond with others. However, if you drink alone or have numerous drinks each day, it may

become a harmful habit. If you can't stop yourself, you can develop an alcohol consumption disorder. Giving up alcohol may allow you to devote more time to your relationships, job, and health. It may also help with despair and anxiety, as well as boost your self-esteem.

Cancer Risks Reduced (Maybe)

It's obvious that alcohol, especially heavy drinking, increases your risk of developing malignancies in your esophagus (food pipe), mouth, throat, and breast. It's less clear whether stopping alcohol reduces your risk of cancer and, if so, how long it takes. Some research points to possible benefits, but scientists aren't convinced.

It's possible that your sex life will improve.

A little booze may make couples more flirtatious. However, consuming more than one drink every day, especially if you abuse or are addicted to alcohol, has the opposite impact. Men may have difficulty obtaining and maintaining an erection. Women's sex drive may decrease, and their vaginal tissues may become drier. Reduce your alcohol consumption and see whether it improves your romance.

You'll Get More Sleep

At first, alcohol may make you sleepy. However, if you fall asleep, it can wake you up several times during the night. It also interferes with your breathing and disturbs the critical REM stage of sleep. You may also need to get up more frequently to pee. For a more pleasant night's sleep, avoid alcohol, especially in the late afternoon and evening.

You'll be less likely to become ill.

Even a single episode of excessive drinking can impair your body's ability to fight germs for up to 24 hours. Large doses of alcohol weaken your immune system and body's ability to restore itself over time. Reduce your alcohol consumption to better protect yourself from disease.

Blood Pressure Control

If you drink a lot and have high blood pressure, you might be able to lower your readings by doing one easy thing: not drinking alcohol. Even cutting back on alcoholic beverages might have a significant impact. Discuss your numbers with your doctor.

Blood pressure should be less than 120/80. If your blood pressure is more than 130/80, you have high blood pressure.

Clear Your Mind

Alcoholism can make it difficult to think and remember things. Heavy drinking can alter your perception of distances and volumes over time, as well as slow down and impair your motor skills. It may even make it more difficult for you to read the emotions of others. However, if you stop smoking, your brain appears to restore some of these talents.

Withdrawal

If you're a heavy drinker, cutting out all alcohol may cause your body to protest at first. You may experience cold sweats, a racing heart, nausea, vomiting, trembling hands, and severe anxiety. Some folks even experience convulsions or have visions of things that aren't there (hallucinations). To help you get through it, your doctor or drug abuse therapist can offer advice and prescribe medications such as benzodiazepines or carbamazepine.

What Happens to Your Body and Brain When You Stop Drinking Alcohol

It doesn't have to be the start of a new year to feel like you need a fresh start, especially if you're trying to kick a bad habit. While there's nothing wrong with the occasional drink, there are many other advantages to going dry that go beyond brighter skin and improved sleep. Soroya Bacchus, M.D., a board-certified psychiatrist specializing in addiction medicine, adds, "The mental health issues are equally as significant as the physical ones." "Both the mood and the cognitive abilities improve." According to the National Institute on Alcohol Abuse and Alcoholism, moderate drinking for women is defined as up to three drinks in 24 hours and a maximum of seven drinks a week.

Here's what you can expect when you stop drinking alcohol, regardless of where you fall on the scale; use this as an encouragement to get started on your resolution before the New Year.

One Day Later

This question's answer is heavily dependant on how many cocktails you had the night before. Day one will most likely be business as usual if you stick to water. On the other hand, if you opted to eat to prepare for your fast, the first day will almost certainly be filled with withdrawal symptoms. As Bacchus explains, alcohol leads the brain to release the feel-good chemical dopamine, which triggers an emotional crash the next

day. Expect psychological indicators like irritation, food cravings, anxiety, and even signs of depression, as well as physical withdrawal symptoms, including restlessness, headaches, thirst, and nausea.

One Week Later

You'll start to feel the mental and emotional benefits after around seven days of abstinence. First and foremost, you'll sleep better, which will result in more energy, a better mood, and greater cognitive performance.

According to the National Sleep Foundation, "while alcohol, a depressant, can help you fall asleep faster, it also contributes to poor-quality sleep later." It can prevent REM sleep, increase respiratory issues, upset your circadian cycle, and cause more frequent nighttime toilet trips. Better-quality sleep can help to reduce mood swings, reduce food cravings, and improve cognitive function, resulting in increased mental clarity and memory.

Alcohol exacerbates pre-existing mental health disorders like anxiety and sadness. Without alcohol and the subsequent hangover, sufferers may feel more emotionally stable and clearheaded. "People typically drink alcohol to unwind because it is a depressive and has a sedative effect," says Meredith Watkins of American Addiction Centers. "However, it can cause anxiety in as little as a few hours after consumption."

One month later

This is when in-depth introspection and long-term lifestyle changes may be required. You may find it easier to maintain a healthy lifestyle without the temptations, sleep deprivation, and mood changes that come with partying and hangovers. You'll have more time to devote to self-care or other interests that used to take a back place to boisterous brunches and wine-fueled dinners, as Bacchus points out. Instead of recovering from a Saturday night out, spend your Sunday trying a new gym class or mastering a difficult cuisine.

Finally, abstaining from alcohol may enable you to

recognize what drinking is concealing (if anything). Bacchus suggests that you ask yourself questions such as: Do I use it to unwind socially? Is it possible that I'm drinking to hide my worry or discomfort? Answering honestly and openly could lead to a more mindful relationship with your evening glass of wine.

What are the Emotional Effects of Alcohol?

Many of us drink to feel joyful or relaxed and hide or escape our emotions. Alcohol is a potent narcotic that can appear to be a one-stop answer to any problem at first. When used carefully, it can even be beneficial. When a person abuses alcohol, however, the emotional consequences it causes can work against them.

In addition to its physiological effects, alcohol has several emotional consequences. In reality, people are often motivated to drink by the emotional changes that alcohol causes. Simply put, when people learn to use alcohol to help them deal with a short- term emotional difficulty, they risk developing a much more significant long-term problem – addiction.

How We Use Alcohol to Manage Emotions

Alcohol is commonly used to induce pleasurable feelings, relieve painful ones, or induce relaxation. It can assist us in expressing our feelings more forcefully or masking those we don't want to convey.

People look for alcohol to celebrate and heighten their happiness when they are joyful. Alcohol can improve confidence and self-esteem in social circumstances, allowing people to bond and have a good time. Alcohol can help shy people relax and enjoy themselves by lowering inhibitions and allowing them to have more fun.

When people are in agony, they turn to alcohol to help them cope with their feelings of despair, pain, embarrassment, and loneliness. It can be used to help people deal with sadness, fear, jealousy, and hopelessness. Alcohol can briefly take people's attention away from the problem. It can make things appear better than they are, even if only for a short while.

When people are worried, they often turn to alcohol for self-medicating. It can assist a person in relaxing, quiet down, and lessen their level of anxiety. Alcohol functions as an emotional numbing agent in these situations. It permits people to avoid rather than intensify their feelings.

And the Effects of Alcohol on Our Emotions

Our brain is affected by alcohol in a variety of ways. Although it affects every portion of the brain, specific areas are particularly affected. The parts of our emotional processing that alcohol effects are all linked to our emotional processing. Alcohol alters brain chemistry by interfering with hormones that regulate our emotions.

Unless someone begins to drink alcohol, these changes are usually just transient. They then tend to linger long after the final drink has been consumed.

This is why some alcoholics appear unstable not only

when they're drinking but also when they're not. They may cry or lash out in frustration. They may also appear manic if they act "too cheerful." After drinking, those who show indicators of alcohol misuse are more prone to feel violent.

Contrary to popular opinion, the sort of alcohol you consume does not affect your mood. Rather, a person's choice of beverage is likely to be influenced by their mood. Or, perhaps, based on preconceived notions, on the mood they desire to be in. For example, one individual might unwind with a glass of red wine after work, while another would calm down with a shot of whiskey when they're agitated. Many people will drink Champagne to make themselves joyful.

Several different factors influence the level to which alcohol affects one's emotions, including:

•Amount eaten

•Use history and duration

•Family history

•Genetic considerations

•Environment

•Psychological issues

•General health

The Negative Effects of Alcohol on Emotional Well-Being

We use alcohol to change our emotions in various ways, so, understandably, an emotional imbalance might lead to alcohol abuse. Unfortunately, drinking can exacerbate bad emotions over time. This can lead to a downward spiral into alcoholism.

Short-Term Effects of Alcohol on Emotions

Alcohol can skew people's perceptions of a situation since it has the ability to enhance emotions. For example, if a drinker sees someone with a little unhappy face, their mind may tend to inflate this into a full-fledged rage.

The effects of alcohol on mood and a lack of inhibition can cause problems for anyone. A person may have social problems due to their unstable behavior, such as getting into fights.

It can also make a person think about self-harm or suicide, especially if they have depressed inclinations.

A person's problems may worsen the next day after drinking, especially if they blacked out. This could be a result of embarrassment or frustration with oneself for acting irrationally. Or they may be remorseful of actions taken as a result of bad judgment.

If someone is hungover and hasn't gotten enough sleep, they may be more sensitive than usual and may get irritated as a result. As a result, if individuals committed blunders the night before, they have the potential to make things considerably worse the next day.

Alcohol's Long-Term Emotional Effects

Although some of the consequences of alcohol are transient and may be overcome, repeated binges that end in guilt and regret can deteriorate your mental health over time. As a result, you may find yourself drinking to cope with the consequences of your actions.

In the long run, brain damage from heavy drinking can wreak havoc on your productivity and memory. This can make you irritated with yourself and undermine your self-esteem over time.

Self-medicating with alcohol can sometimes lead to isolation. This could be due to lost relationships or embarrassment about your poor coping skills. Depression and other bad emotions can be exacerbated by isolation. Furthermore, you are more likely to begin drinking alone, which might have a more negative emotional impact than drinking with others.

Alcohol was more likely to cause emotional shifts in social drinkers. These emotions were mostly positive because alcohol acted as a source of connection. On the other hand,

Solo drinkers were less likely to gain from the emotional impact and were more likely to just experience physiological changes.

When alcohol abuse is involved, the effects of alcohol on emotion might last for a long time. Another study indicated that even after a person has detoxed, heavy drinking might contribute to emotional instability. After a long duration of drinking, an alcoholic's brain is likely to demonstrate decreased emotion perception, even when sober.

Alcohol and Mental Health

Alcoholism has long been linked to co-morbid mental diseases. Many persons who suffer from anxiety, depression, schizophrenia, or mood disorders self-medicate with alcohol. Alcohol and drug misuse, on the other hand, can cause or exacerbate these problems.

Alcohol can be used to temporarily ease the unpleasant symptoms associated with sadness and anxiety. Long-term alcohol consumption, on the other hand, tends to exacerbate them in both circumstances. Furthermore, alcohol might be a trigger if a person is susceptible to depression or anxiety but does not have it.

Alcohol is known to cause depressive episodes in bipolar people. Drinking can make those with mood disorders feel even more unstable.

Of course, if someone uses alcohol as a form of emotional support regularly, they may develop alcoholism.

Alcohol Isn't a Solution Outside of Chemistry

While alcohol might enhance our emotional well-being, it can also delete it. While it is acceptable to drink in moderation in every scenario, it should not be misused. You may have a problem if you find yourself reaching for a drink frequently, whether you are pleased, furious, or depressed.

People who use alcohol as a kind of self-medication are in danger of becoming addicted.

In addition to the drinking, it is critical to treat any underlying emotional or psychological disorders during rehabilitation. If you have been diagnosed with or are at

risk of developing a mental health problem, you should seek treatment in a facility that specializes in dual diagnosis.

It might take years to recover from psychological harm caused or exacerbated by drinking, so it's critical to get the right help and support.

These are the 12 steps I took to quit drinking and stay sober. When I first wake up in the morning, I take a few moments to appreciate the sensation of being sober.

I never get tired of saying "thanks to being free" first thing in the morning. Every day, I appreciate my higher powers for providing me the strength to be sober. I also give myself credit for the hard work I'm putting in to overcome my addiction.

I once read that sobriety is similar to deodorant in that it must be applied every day to be effective!

2.In the beginning, I used relaxing and healing pills and herbs from the health food store.

Lemon balm, kava, chamomile, valerian, lavender, and passionflower are added to the vitamin B complex. I also utilized the herb kudzu to calm my appetite. Perhaps it was the placebo effect, but it seemed to work for me. I drank lots of herbal tea as well.

3.I visited a few blogs in the morning and evening to see how folks were doing.

I used to read Belle's blog, Soberistas, and Mrs. D's blog, among others, but they're no longer live. I didn't discover the Boom Community until I had been on the site for over a year. Of all the blogs I've read in the last few years, Boom is by far my favorite.

4.I read a lot of stop fiction and books on the science of recovery!

William Porter's Alcohol Explained was a game-changer for me. However, there are a plethora of fantastic options. There are numerous methods to sobriety.

Every book I read taught me something.

I realized I was going through FAB after reading Alcohol Explained (fading affect bias). Humans, according to William Porter's brilliant book, forget unpleasant experiences faster than joyful ones. As a result, I'm going to refresh my memories   I recall the excruciating headaches, hours of vomiting, self-loathing, missing crucial events because I was too hungover, looking like a jerk, and not having the stamina to care for myself or the house before I stopped drinking.

It was neither enjoyable nor restful. It was a living horror.

5.When I had cravings, I ate many foods that I wouldn't have allowed myself to eat if I hadn't been drinking because of the calories.

I gave myself a lot of sober rewards. I was also constantly stuffing olives and little Reese's peanut butter cups into my mouth! Nutella was eaten straight from the jar. I even drank a shot of olive brine to jolt myself out of severe hunger. It was successful!

Thankfully, that time is passed. I don't get cravings very often anymore, and when I do, they're only for a short time.

6.I go for a lot of alone walks to contemplate and clear

my head.

7.I discovered the benefits of meditation. I now meditate regularly.

8.I drew clear lines on the sand.

People had come to expect me to be a people pleaser. I felt bad about drinking all the time, so I attempted to be everything to everyone. That had to come to an end. It's not always easy, but I remind myself to put on my oxygen mask first.

similar material to read

9.I started a hobby to divert my attention away from drinking.

10.I registered for a few classes.

Because I had to drive, going to class kept me sober and provided me something to do on the nights when I would have been drinking.

11.I don't think about it very frequently, but I remember some of the truly horrible occasions when I was drinking.

I recall some of the horrible things I did and tell my

friends about them; I don't want to linger on them, but I also don't want to forget them. I don't want to lapse into a state of sober complacency and believe I wasn't as horrible as I thought. I keep reminding myself that, sure, I was that horrible. I was genuinely on my knees a year ago, hungover once more. My self-hatred is at an all-time high. I couldn't wait for it to be over. I was so depressed that I prayed to my higher powers for the strength to get sober and stop hating myself. It's important to note that interacting with my higher powers or praying were unique experiences for me. It was not something I did regularly. However, I was desperate and had run out of options for stopping the madness."

12.I consider how far my life has progressed.

I remind myself of all the things for which I am grateful. I'm thankful I was able to stop drinking alcohol before it became more appealing than life itself.

I was reading numerous blogs that appeared to have had a sour ending for the authors. When I think of such blogs, I become a little scared. The two bloggers that had the most impact on me were two humorous, charming, and intelligent women who appeared to have overcome their addictions. Because I was still battling in the early days, I recall being slightly envious of their sobriety. They both relapsed after more than a year of sobriety, and neither was able to find their way back to sobriety. One attempted suicide, while the other frequently tweeted about their mental suffering because they drank again, only to disappear.

I imagine them happily sober and too preoccupied to post on occasion. But I have a sneaking suspicion that this isn't the case. And that saddens and frightens me enough to stay clean because I know my tale would end badly if I started drinking again.

After all, alcohol is addictive, and you will get addicted if you consume enough of it. Addictions can and do kill people.

CONCLUSION

Alcoholism is when, given its detrimental effects, one can no longer regulate alcohol consumption, compulsively misuse alcohol, and/or suffer mental distress while not drinking.

To quit drinking, using hypnosis is a realistic choice for those who want to change their lives.

Alcoholism is an illness that causes millions of deaths each year. Thousands of people around the world are succumbing to the consequences and every day suffering from alcohol poisoning. More than 15 million people are estimated to be dealing with alcoholism in the USA alone. The numbers are very troubling.

For decades now, people have viewed hypnosis as an effective treatment choice for substance use disorders. We also know that hypnosis can motivate abusers to give up alcohol due to clinical research and can even avoid relapses.

Why are people addicted to alcohol? What makes men and women worldwide drink into oblivion?

Alcohol functions as a central nervous system

depressant which means alcohol intake reduces normal brain function. Through the activity of a neurotransmitter called GABA (or gamma-aminobutyric acid), alcohol helps to slow the brain. On top of this, alcohol also interacts with natural endorphin production.

How GABA Changes Your Brain

GABA is the neurotransmitter responsible for your brain's inhibitions which makes it non-specific. The neurotransmitter does not reach a particular part of the brain when the GABA signals are increased but affects all of it instead. This is why people who drink heavily show symptoms such as poor motor control (have difficulty walking), loss of memory, impaired verbal skills (slurred speech), or even loss of consciousness.

Nonetheless, here's the crunch. Your body can adapt to its environment, and the brain is possibly the first to adapt to every scenario. When you drink alcohol regularly, the brain can adjust to tolerate GABA 's inhibitory effects by increasing the stimulating effects of other neurotransmitters such as glutamate.

There are opposing effects of glutamate and GABA. Your body relies on glutamate to transmit signals at an increased rate when the brain needs to. Yet to survive GABA's inhibitive effects, the body is changing to produce more glutamate.

As a result, you grow a tolerance for alcohol. Alcohol induces the same effects in your body, but you're more immune to its inhibitory effects. And, to get into the same state of drunkenness, you need to drink more.

Your body adjusting to GABA is the start of a vicious tolerance circle – increased drinking – greater tolerance – even more drinking, and so on. Finally, the vicious cycle contributes to dependency and addiction.

The Dark Side of Alcohol Tolerance

And if you thought this was the story's ending, you were mistaken. The brain adapts to withstand GABA's inhibitive effects by increasing glutamate production. But when this happens, when you stop drinking, you will start having withdrawal symptoms such as tremors (usually in the hands), hallucinations, and even convulsions.

That is because your brain is over-stimulated now. The brain has evolved to send further signals to surmount GABA's inhibitive effects and will continue to do so even though you quit drinking for a while.

If you've hit that level, it's fair to say you're into alcohol addiction. It would be very difficult to leave, and it may be risky to stop drinking altogether.

How Alcohol Interferes with Endorphins

Alcohol helps the body release more endorphins. Endorphins are naturally occurring substances in your body that act as neurotransmitters and send signals from one neuron to another. Your body has more than 20 forms of endorphins, and beta-endorphins have greater effects than cocaine or even morphine.

By now, you've already read of dopamine, oxytocin, and serotonin. Okay, these molecules are endorphins, and they are involved in many processes, ranging from producing euphoria and calming feelings to supporting women during conception.

Recent studies indicate that alcohol does affect the function of the human brain by inducing the release of endorphins. It is particularly noticeable in those who began to drink alcohol as adolescents.

And you can feel how alcohol contributes to endorphin release.

•You feel comfortable as soon as you have a drink, or you might even be feeling euphoric.

•Your inhibitions are dropping along with your other brain functions-making you feel confident and capable.

•Not only are your inhibitions reduced, but the logical part of your brain is impaired, and you are susceptible to make decisions that have potentially negative or dangerous consequences.

•Alcohol is relaxing your mind and body, so you can feel like getting a couple before you go to bed. It can cause you to believe you are unable to sleep without alcohol consumption, leading to the development of mental barriers that hamper your attempts to give up booze.